Wild Food Identification Guide

by Linda Runyon

A Wild Food Company Publication

Wild Food Identification Guide
November 2011

Published by
the Wild Food Company
Dorchester, Massachusetts

DISCLAIMER

This book is intended to be an educational tool for identifying the wild foods that are highlighted in Linda Runyon's *The Essential Wild Food Survival Guide*. The information presented is for use as a supplement to a healthy, well-rounded lifestyle. The nutritional requirements of individuals may vary greatly, therefore the author and publisher take no responsibility for an individual using and ingesting wild food.

There are many variations of plants and the additional danger of poisionous look-alikes; as such, all responsibility lies with the forager. Do not rely on any one reference, but rather use several good references. The author finds this reference adequate from her experience, but you must develop your own research, observations and experience.

State and local regulations on foraging vary, but mostly there are re- strictions against taking wild food from public land. You should always check with park officials before foraging anywhere but on your own land. If you know you are, or might be, on private land and wish to forage there, be sure to get the land owner's permission to do so.

ISBN 978-0-936699-27-1

Printed in the United States of America

OfTheField.com

The Wild Food Company
101 Train Street, Suite 1
Dorchester, MA 02122

Other Wild Food Survival Materials by Linda Runyon

The Essential Wild Food Survival Guide

Linda Runyon's Master Class on Wild Food Survival DVD

Eat the Trees!

Wild Cards

A Survival Acre

Homestead Memories

Why Not LOVE?

Wild Food & Animals Coloring Book

Basic Middle Eastern Desert Survival Guide

PHOTOGRAPHY

Thanks for photographs from
Ruth Demers, Eric Conover,
Paul Runyon, Jr., Kerin A. Denser-Fuzy
and Chris Parfitt

ACKNOWLEDGMENTS

Thanks to Rosary Shepherd for layout, editing and typesetting, and my son Eric for cover design and image handling. This wouldn't have been possible without you both! Thanks also to Steve Arnold and Ann Pedrick.

Linda Runyon

TABLE OF CONTENTS

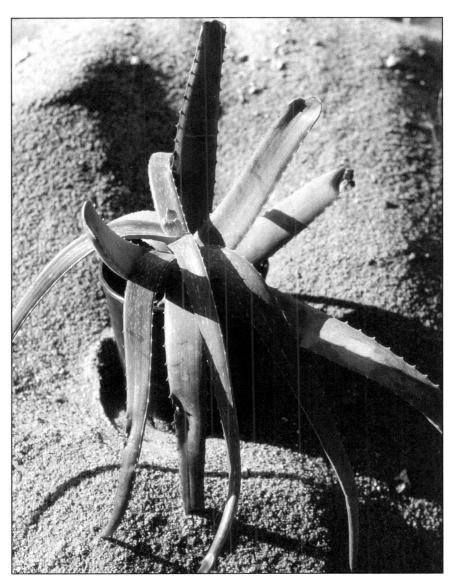

Aloe Vera

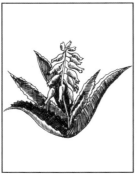

Habitat: Temperate zones, desert, arid regions.

Characteristics: Green succulent leaves, called spikes, are filled with clear gel. Mature plant has spikes up to 3' high with dense, arrow-shaped clusters of yellow or orange flowers.

1

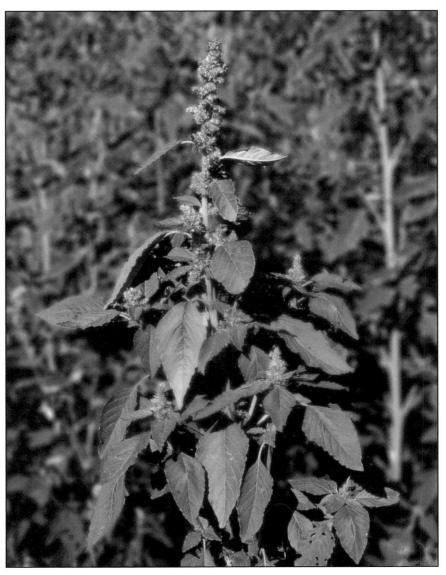

Amaranth

Habitat: Cultivated soil.

Characteristics: Height 2' but could be as tall as 6'. Has bristly seed heads clustered on multi-branch stems from a central stalk. Seeds are black and shiny, leaves are smooth and veined with slightly toothed margins.

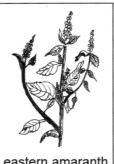

eastern amaranth

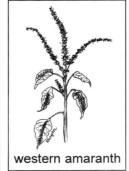

western amaranth

2

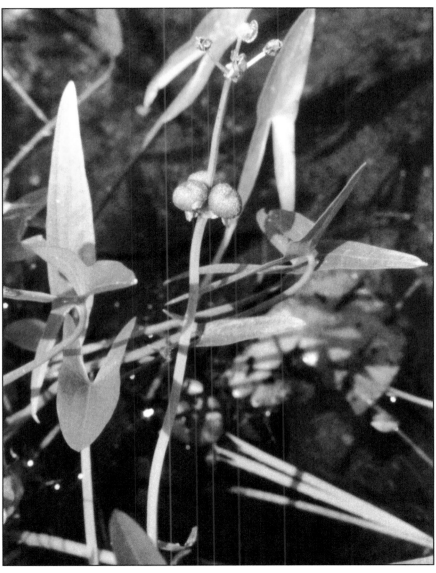

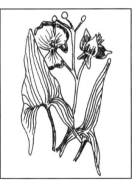

Arrowhead

Habitat: Widely distributed: marshes, wet bogs, mud flats.

Characteristics: Grows in swamp water to a height of 10" or more. Arrowhead-shaped leaves, white, four-petal, filmy flowers.

Warning: Food purity is as clean as the water it grows in. Harvest from clean waters only.

3

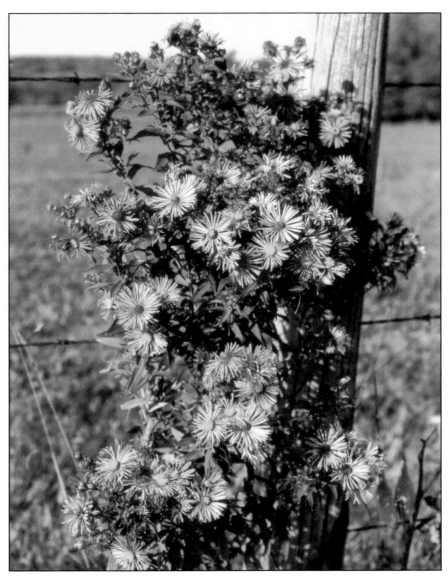

Aster

Habitat: Fields and meadows, roadsides.

Characteristics: Height averages 24", may reach to 40" or higher. Numerous extensions jutting with multi-petaled flowers from central stem. Petals layered in flat, 1/2"-long sections; colors include white, pink, yellow, blue, purple.

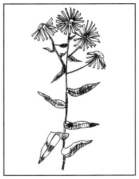

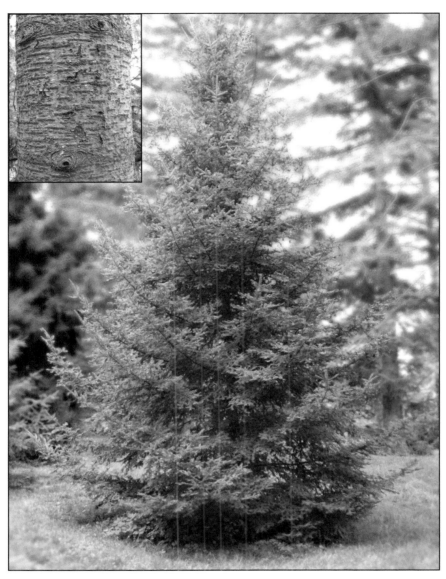

Balsam Fir

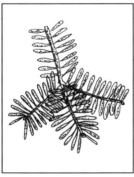

Habitat: Cool, moist, acidic soil along roadsides, woods or lawns and in softwood forests.

Characteristics: Tree has small, short needles growing alternatively from under stem, 1" to 1 1/2" long. Grows to height of 40' to 60'. Bark is ash-grey, relatively smooth, and has blisters filled with sap. (Large trunk pictured.)

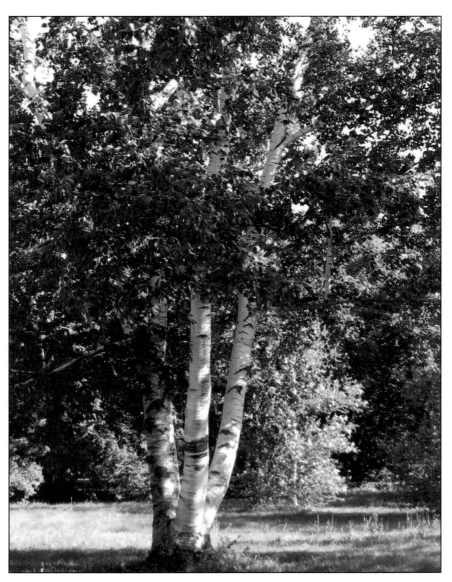

Birch

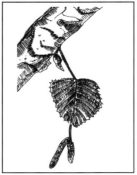

Habitat: Woods, roadsides.

Characteristics: Alternate, simple, saw-toothed leaves. Papery bark of the white and yellow birch peels in curls.

CAUTION: Do not peel outer skin as this could kill the tree.

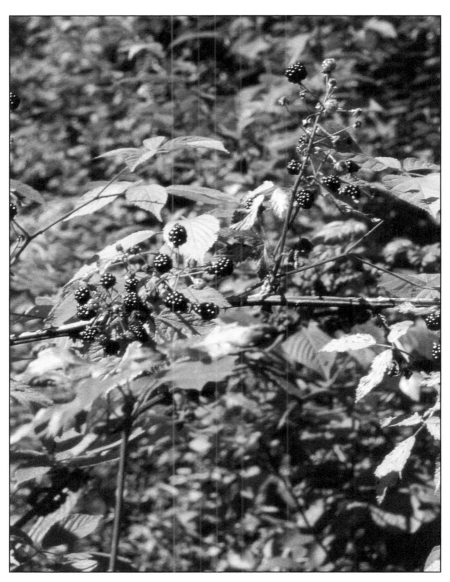

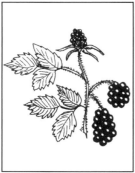

Blackberry

Habitat: Roadsides, fields, meadows.

Characteristics: Bush varies in size, up to 5' or 6' tall. Saw-toothed leaves in groups of 3 to 5; prickers on angular, arching stem. Fruit pebbly and black when ripe.

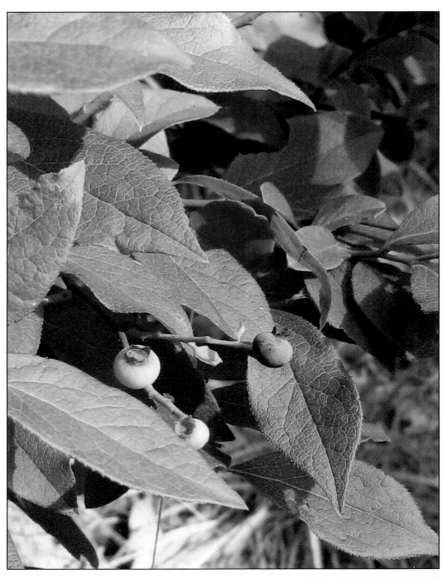

Blueberry

<u>Habitat</u>: Acid soil, fields, roadsides, waste areas, bogs, marshes, woods.

<u>Characteristics</u>: Many varities, from low shrubs to high bushes. Fruit is blue and clusters in groups of 2 to 10. Can identify by characteristic blueberry smell.

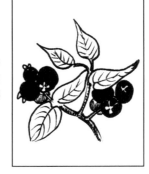

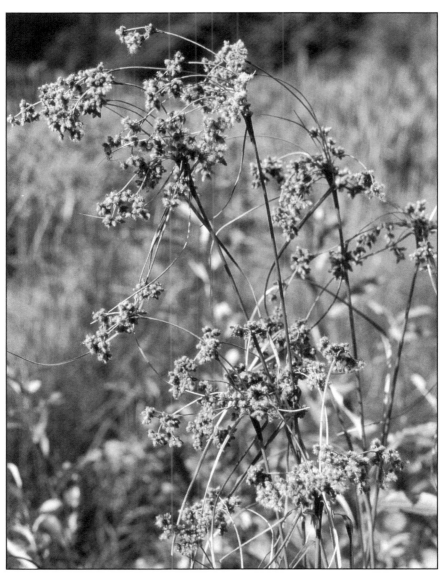

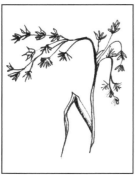

Bulrush

<u>Habitat</u>: Wet areas, drainage spots, bogs, swamps, alongside waterways and ocean bays.

<u>Characteristics</u>: Grasslike herb, many varities. Height 24" or more. Stems smooth, round, with pith. Head of flower spike full of seeds and pollen.

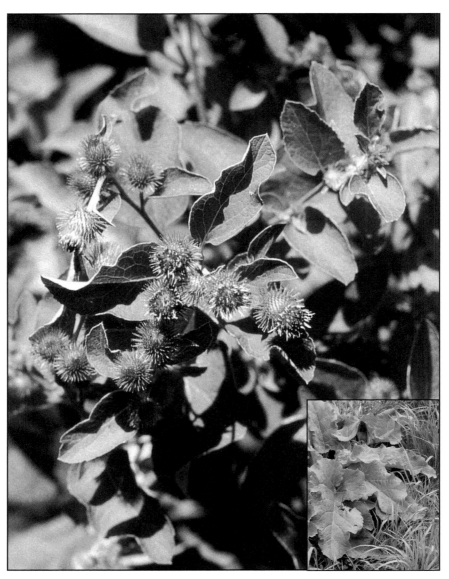

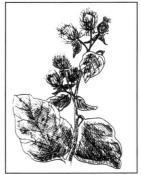

Burdock

<u>Habitat</u>: Fields, roads, most waste areas.

<u>Characteristics</u>: Mature plant has enormous leaves up to 2' wide. Multi-branched stem up to 5' high, has clusters of round burs with bristles.

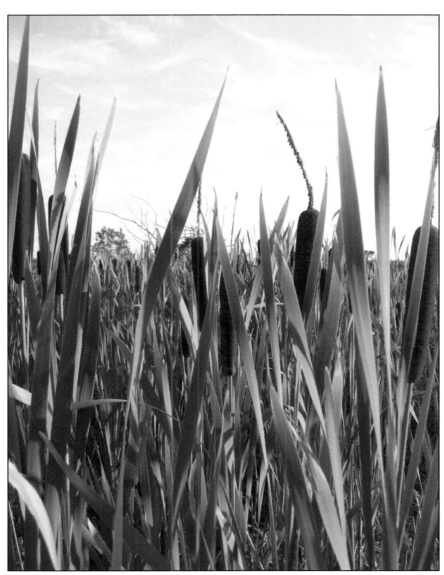

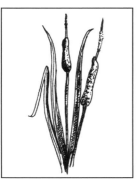

Cattail

Habitat: Bogs, swamps, wet areas.

Characteristics: Grows in wet areas. Height 3' or more. Stalks have hot dog-shaped heads, pollen flags in early spring. The one-veined leaves are very tall and slender.

Warning: Food purity is as clean as the water it grows in. Harvest from clean waters only.

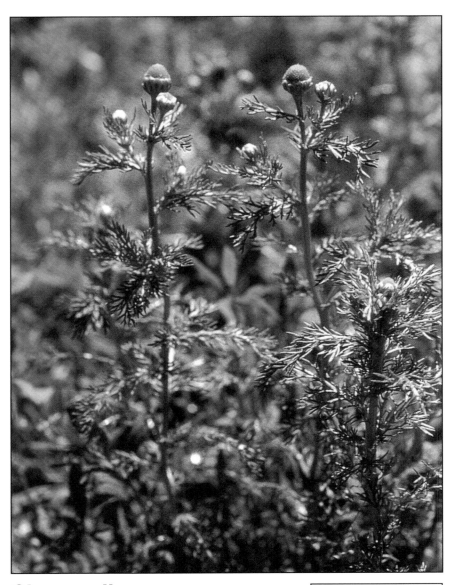

Chamomile

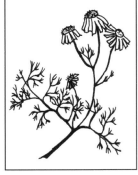

Habitat: Roadsides, "people places", walkways, gardens.

Characteristics: Height averages 3", may reach 12" or more. Has tiny yellow, tight-budded flowers, sweet, pineapple-like smell.

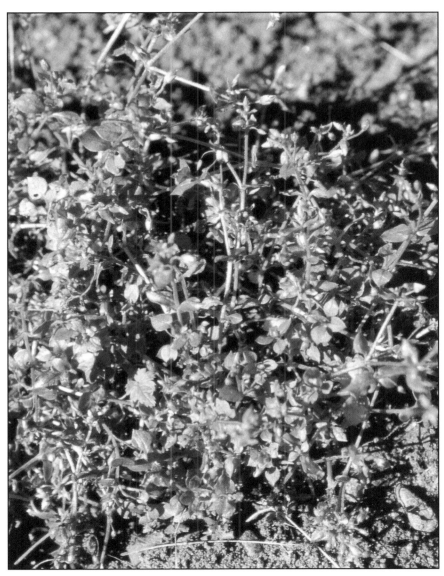

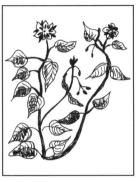

Chickweed

Habitat: Fields, lawns, roadsides, waste places.

Characteristics: Height averages 1" or more; creeps on ground, mats in garden. Tiny paired opposite leaves are ovate and smooth. Star-like white flowers have 5 pairs of petals.

13

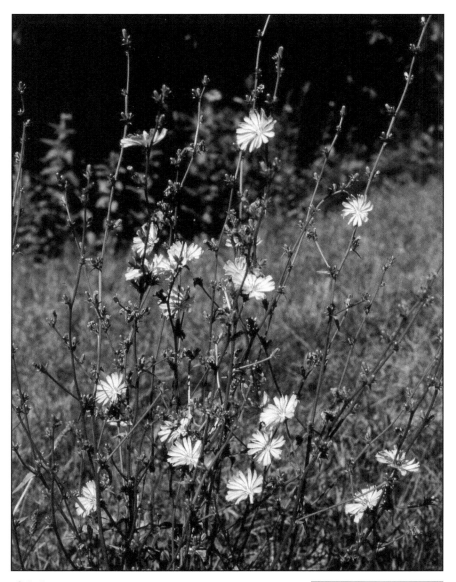

Chicory

<u>Habitat</u>: Roadsides, fields, dry sandy areas.

<u>Characteristics</u>: Height 2' or more. Red-veined, deep-cleft leaves, stem has many star-blue ray flowers.

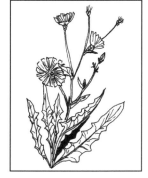

14

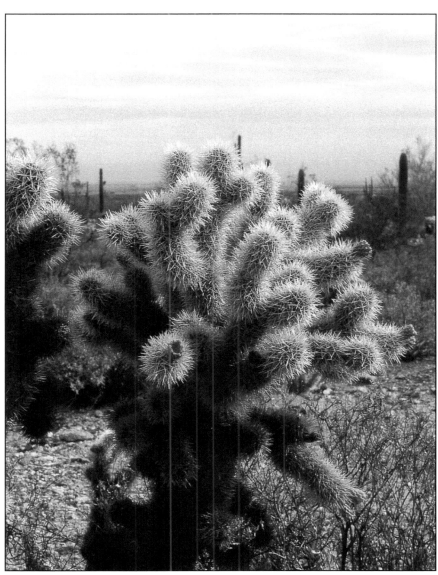

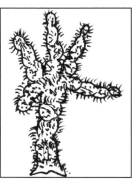

Cholla

Habitat: Desert.

Characteristics: Height 3' to 7' or more. Tree-like cactus, black trunk, thick green stems 3" to 10"; 6-8 silver, barbed spines from each areole. Flower is a light rose color.

WARNING: Use thick gloves; do not touch with bare skin. Spines can penetrate skin, causing vicious stinging and burning.

15

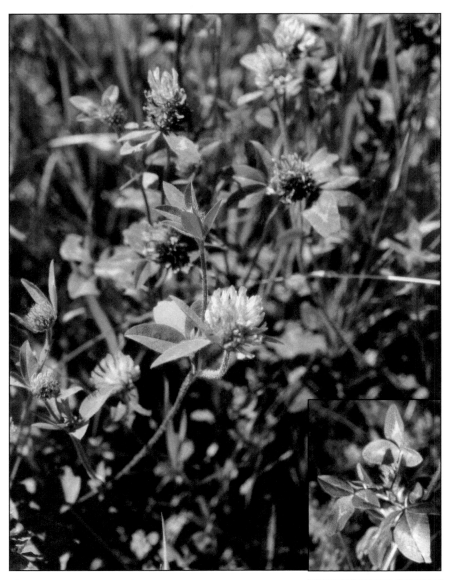

Clover - Red

<u>Habitat</u>: Roadsides, fields, lawns.

<u>Characteristics</u>: Height 10" or more, with hairy stems. Red or purple blossoms with oval nectar sections. Elongated leaves form trefoil with white "V" when mature.

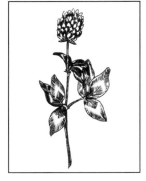

16

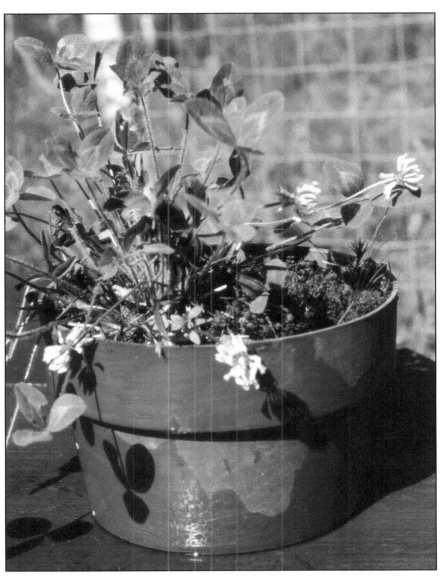

Clover - White

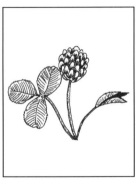

Habitat: Roadsides, fields, lawns.

Characteristics: Height 2" or more. White blossoms have dozens of nectar-filled sections. Round leaves form trefoil at end of stem.

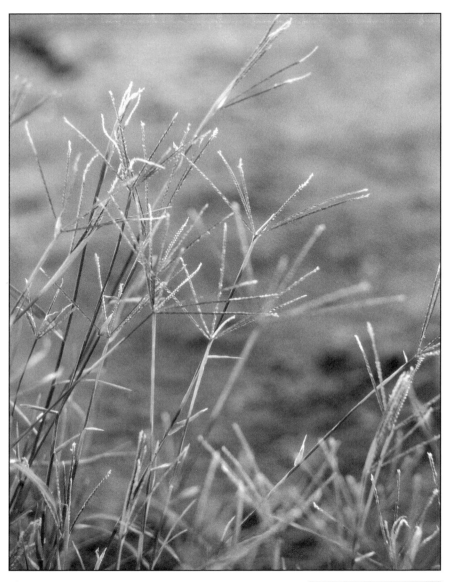

Crabgrass

<u>Habitat</u>: Lawns, roadsides, edges of fields, waste places.

<u>Characteristics</u>: Grass-like; many varieties reaching heights from 3" to 24" or more. Seed tips may vary in amount and thickness.

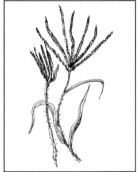

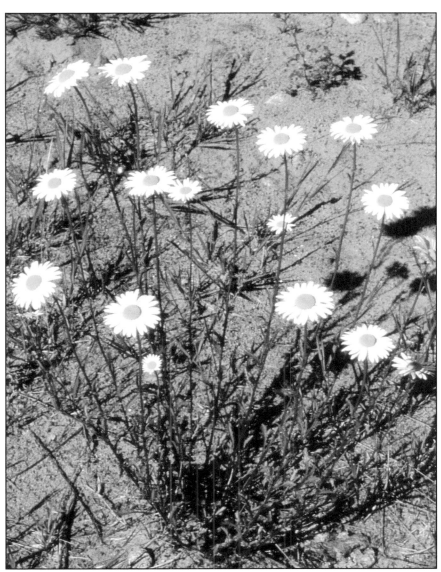

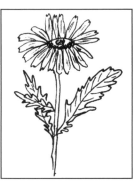

Daisy

Habitat: Lawns, roadsides, fields, waste places.

Characteristics: Height 2' or more; alternate, narrow leaves are clefted and deeply scalloped. White, rayed flower petals, center has a yellow pebbly disk of seeds.

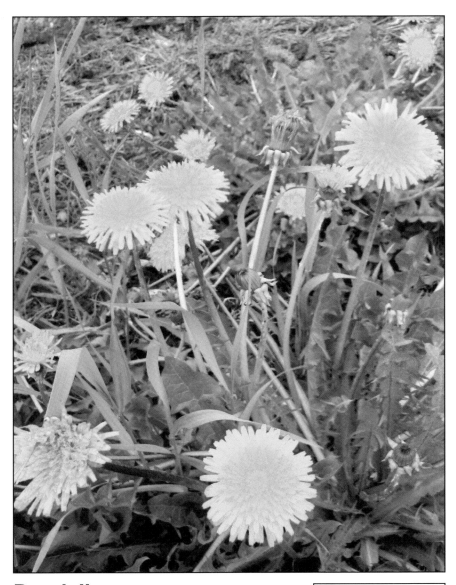

Dandelion

<u>Habitat</u>: Moist areas, lawns, roadsides, fields.

<u>Characteristics</u>: Height 2" or more. Leaves saw-toothed, whorl from center. Leaves and stems show a bit of "milk" when broken. Yellow sectioned flowers mature into fluffy "pompoms" with seeds that blow in the wind.

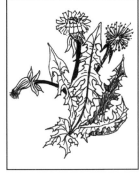

20

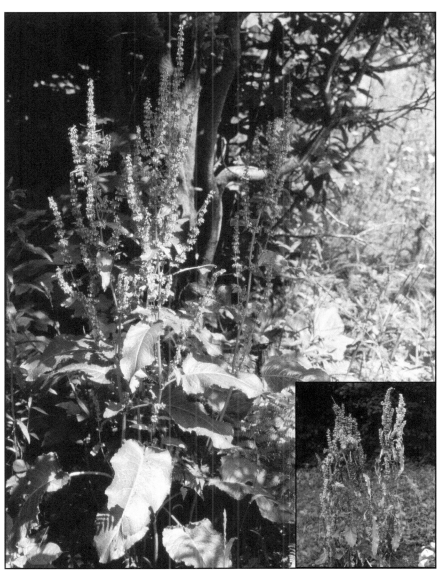

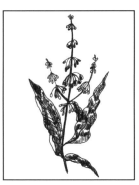

Dock

Habitat: Rich soil, roadsides, fields.

Characteristics: Height 14" or more, clumped. Elongated leaves curl, seeds turn dark brown when dry.

21

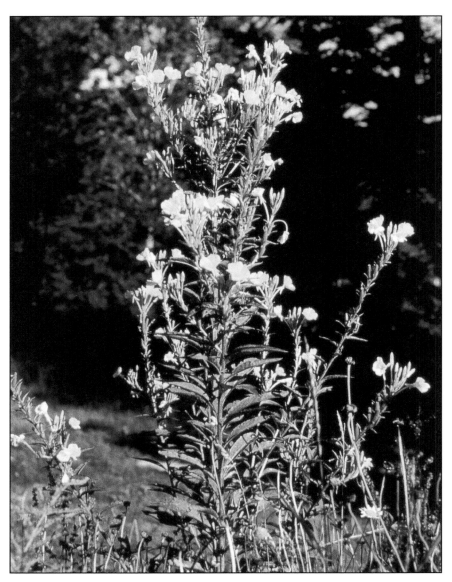

Evening Primrose

<u>Habitat</u>: Gravelly, dry soil, roadsides, waste areas.

<u>Characteristics</u>: Height 2', can reach 5' or more. Long, narrow leaves whorl around center spike-like, hairy stem. Bright yellow flowers have 4 petals, rose-like shape.

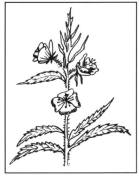

22

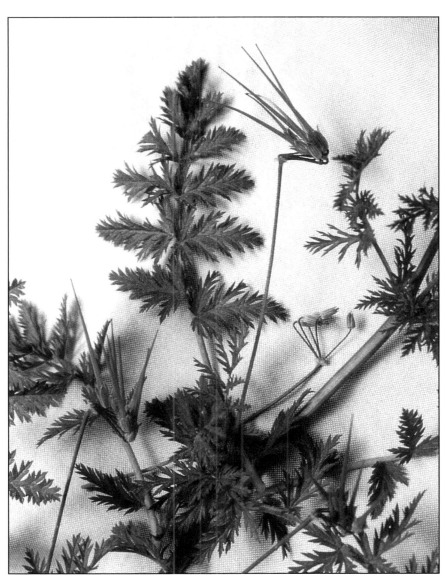

Filaree

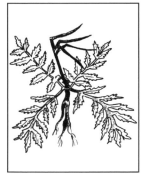

Habitat: Dry areas, desert areas with a little moisture, particularly clay soils.

Characteristics: Height 4" to 20"; stork-bill shaped shoots. Purple flowers on long stalks shoot up from fern-like leaves lying in thick mats. Minute hair on stalks and stems. Leaves produce a celery-like smell when crushed.

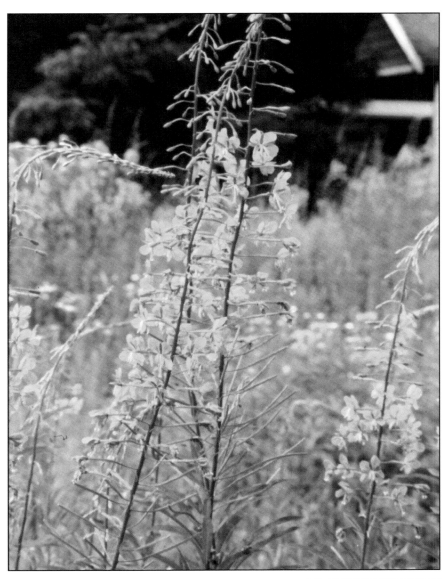

Fireweed

<u>Habitat</u>: Areas where there has been fire, waste areas, areas of regrowth, roadsides, fields.

<u>Characteristics</u>: Height 2' or more. Spike of magenta or pink 4-petaled flowers; elongated top of buds.

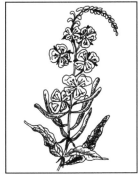

24

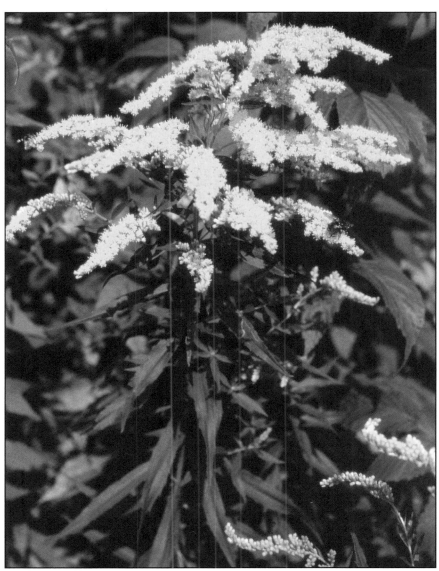

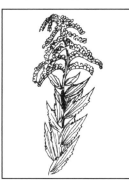

Goldenrod

Habitat: Dry, open fields, woods, road banks, pine barrens, acidic soil.

Characteristics: Height 2' or more. Fluffy, yellow flowers, hundreds of tiny stars on top stalk. The flowers of some species smell like anise.

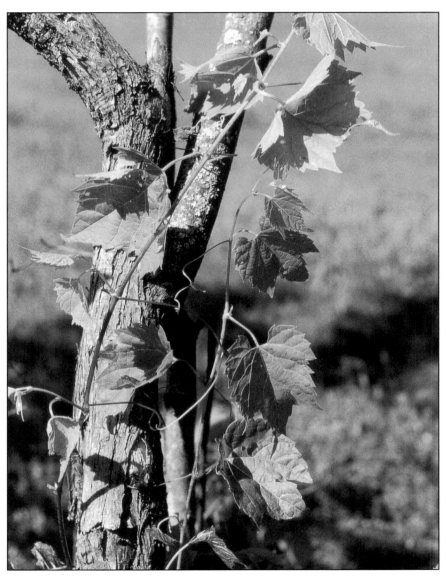

Grape

Habitat: Thickets, edges of woods.

Characteristics: Broad, saw-toothed, heart-shaped leaves, occasional tendrils. Fruits are smaller than commercial grapes and hang in bunches, often black or purple but may vary.

WARNING: LEAVES, FRUIT ARE SIMILAR TO POISONOUS LOOK-ALIKE MOONSEED. Look for wild grape's characteristic red tendrils and saw-toothed leaves; smell for grape odor.

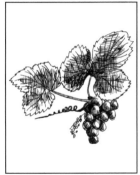

26

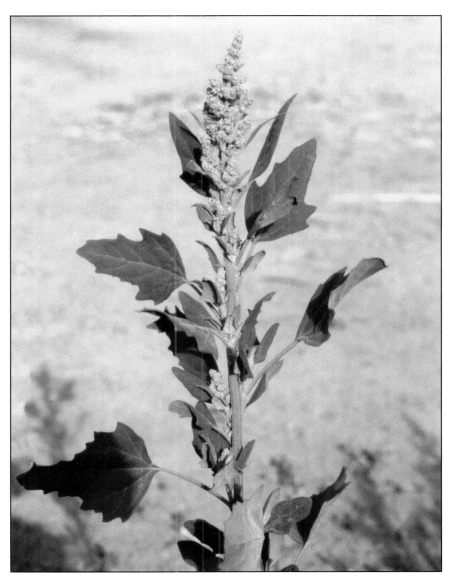

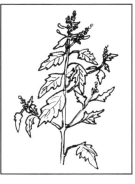

Lamb's Quarters

Habitat: Anywhere weeds grow.

Characteristics: Height 18" or more. Leaf shaped like goose foot and is dark green with whitish underleaf. New leaves have white or lavender-tinged powder near center whorl; seed-like flower clusters are green.

WARNING: LEAF RESEMBLES POISONOUS LOOK-ALIKE NETTLE LEAF GOOSEFOOT, which smells rank. Identify edible plant carefully.

27

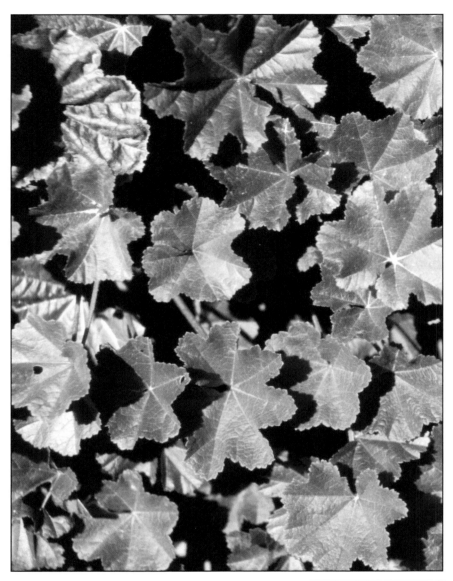

Malva

Habitat: Fields, roadsides, waste areas.

Characteristics: Height 4", may reach to 14". Leaves are circular and shallow-lobed. Seeds are cheese-shaped discs, flowers are 5-petaled in white, pink, or lavender, with a notch at the end of each petal.

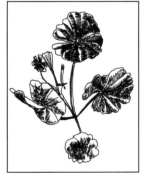

28

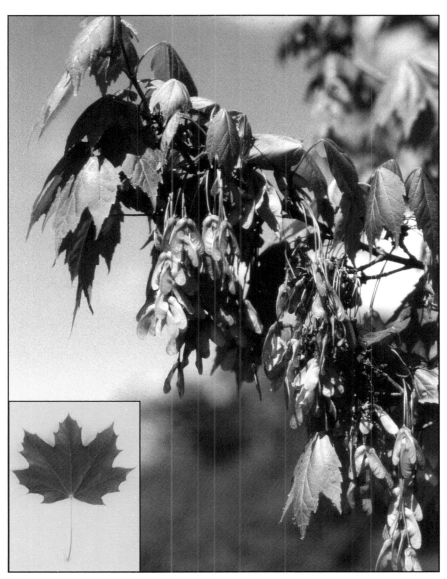

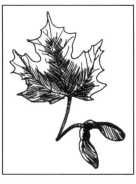

Maple

Habitat: Areas with rich, well-drained soil.

Characteristics: Serrated, deep-lobed, 3-sectioned leaf with definitive points. Bark is dark gray and ranges from smooth to rough. Leaves turn golden yellow to scarlet in early fall. Seeds have brown wings and occur in pairs.

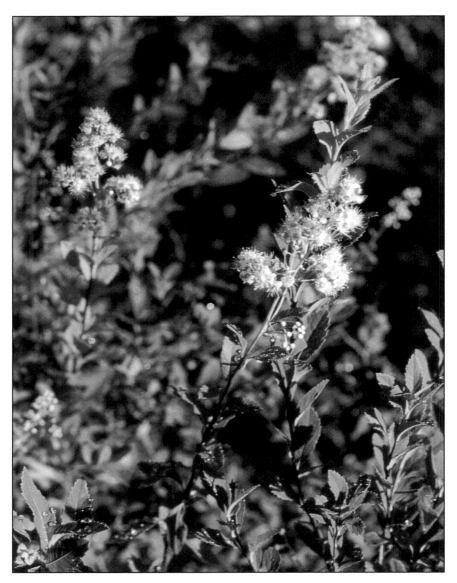

Meadowsweet

Habitat: Meadows, old pastures.

Characteristics: Bush has symmetrical branches 30" long or more. Flower spires, shaped like a church steeple, are white and fluffy in the spring, chocolate brown after maturity in winter.

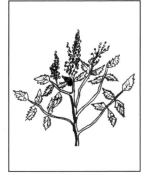

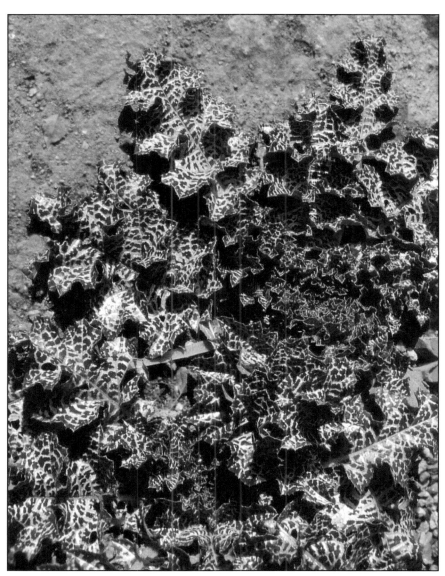

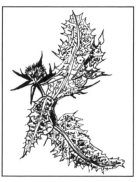

Milk Thistle

Habitat: In west, commonly found in ditches, waste places.

Characteristics: Stalk height is 3' to 6' tall, and leaves can be up to 24" long. White milky splotches on prickly leaves; large, prickly, fuzzy thistle flower with long prickers from central stem.

31

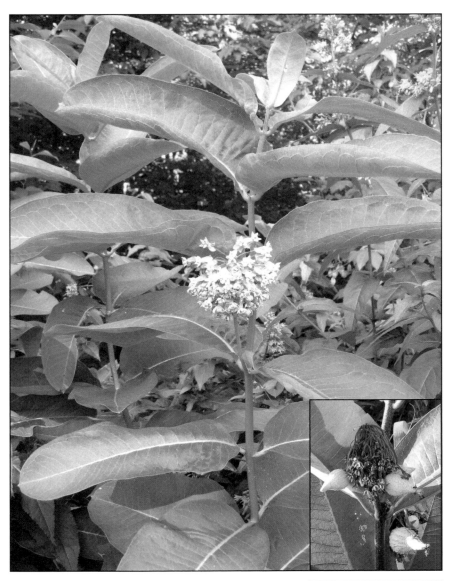

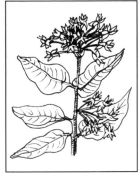

Milkweed

<u>Habitat</u>: Fields, roadsides, gardens.

<u>Characteristics</u>: Height 24" or more. All parts exude a milky sap when broken. Many-clustered flower, white to deep pink; pebbly buds. Tear drop shaped green pod appears after the flower.

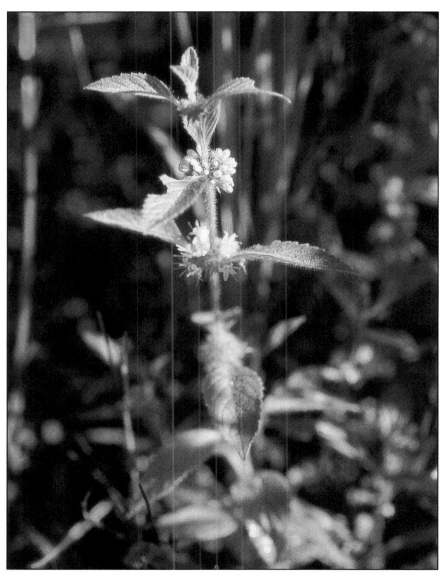

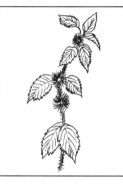

Mint

Habitat: Found in most areas, from swamps to fields, gardens to lawns.

Characteristics: Height can range from 5" to 2'. All varieties have the aromatic minty smell. Stems are square, opposite leaf pairs alternate with saw-toothed edge and prominent veins. Leaves may be smooth or coarse.

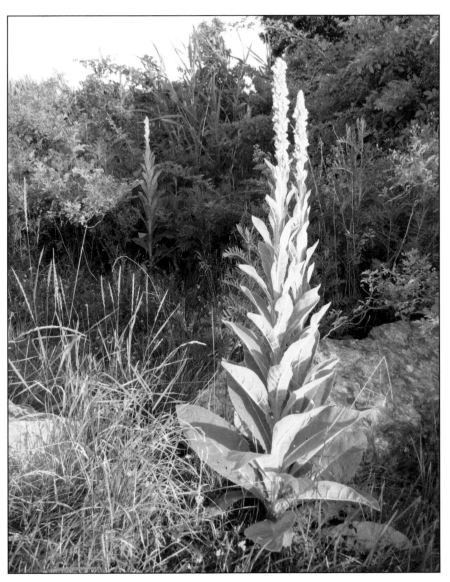

Mullein

Habitat: Waste, wet areas as well as roadsides, gravel-filled fields.

Characteristics: Height 2' or more, can grow up to 10'. Tall spike with small yellow flowers, furry or velvety leaves from 3" to 2' long.

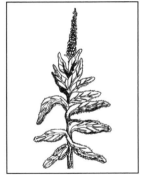

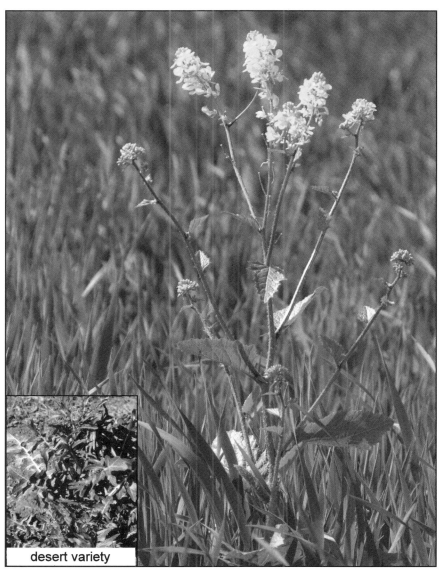

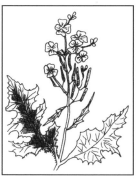

desert variety

Mustard

Habitat: Fields, roadsides in cooler regions.

Characteristics: Height 10" or more. 4-petaled yellow flower, petals in form of a cross; black seeds in pod. Crushed leaf yields herby, pungent smell.

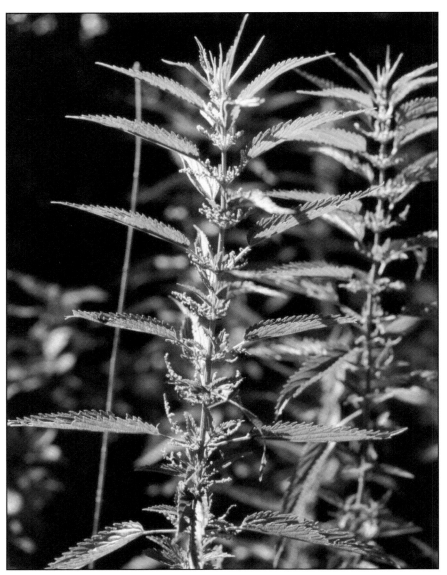

Nettles

Habitat: Fields, fertile soil.

Characteristics: Height 2' or more; erect stalk with numerous branches. Opposite, course, saw-toothed leaves are narrow and broad, seed "chains" in branch intersections.

WARNING: Use gloves, do not touch with bare skin. All parts contain tiny hairs that easily dislodge and can cause stinging, redness, and blisters.

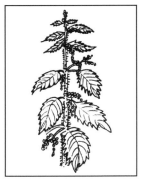

36

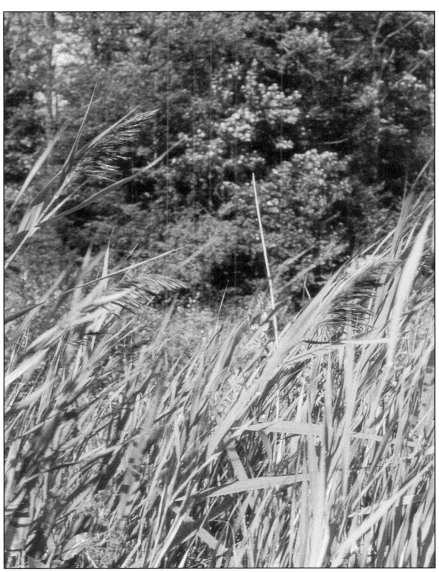

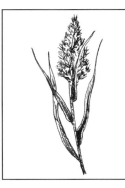

Phragmities

Habitat: Marshes, swamps, wet areas, roadsides.

Characteristics: Height 2' or more, usually 6-8'. Tall, reed-like stalks with feathery seed tips.

Warning: Food purity is as clean as the water it grows in. Harvest from clean waters only.

37

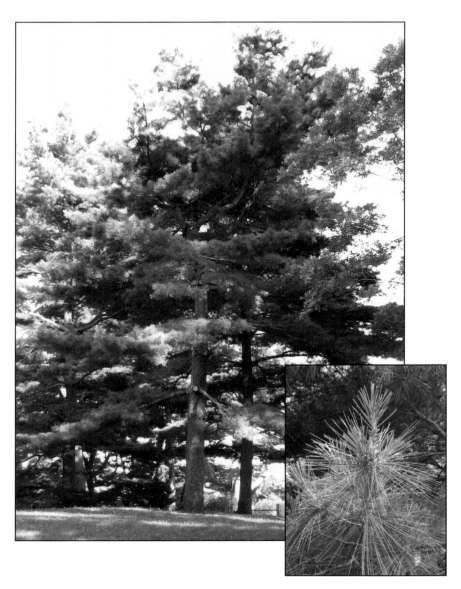

Pine

Habitat: Woods, forests.

Characteristics: Pine trees can grow to a height of 50' or more. The tree has needles instead of leaves, and the outer bark is smooth to scaly. Needles are bundled together, usually in clusters of 2 to 5. The inset photo shows catkins.

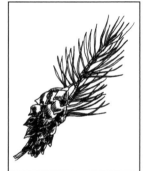

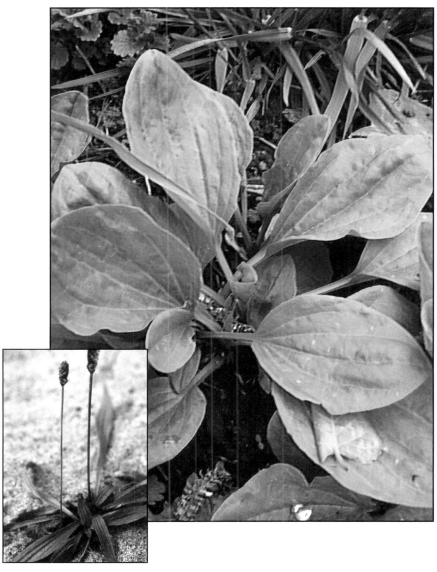

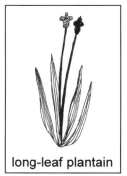

long-leaf plantain

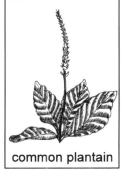

common plantain

Plantain

Habitat: Lawns, roadsides, fields, waste areas.

Characteristics: Both types have heavy-veined leaves and center spikes with seeds. Common plantain has short, broad leaves 2" to 8"; long-leaf plantain has a narrow leaf 10" or more.

39

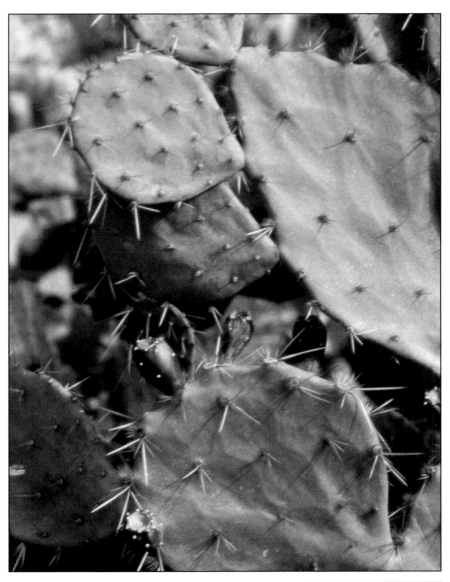

Prickly Pear

<u>Habitat</u>: Hot, dry, well-drained soil.

<u>Characteristics</u>: Fleshy, low-spreading cactus with spiny, thorny, bulb fruit. Pads are roundish and joined.

<u>WARNING</u>: Avoid thorns. Handle pads with extreme care.

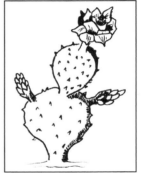

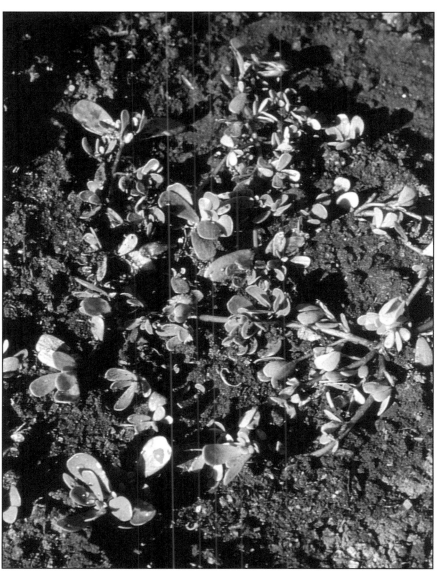

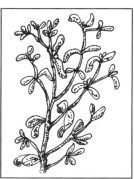

Purslane

Habitat: Fertile soil, topsoil.

Characteristics: Height 1" or more, creeps on ground, makes mats in gardens. Flat-lobed, rounded leaf, oval in shape; 5 to 7 petaled, tiny yellow or red flowers.

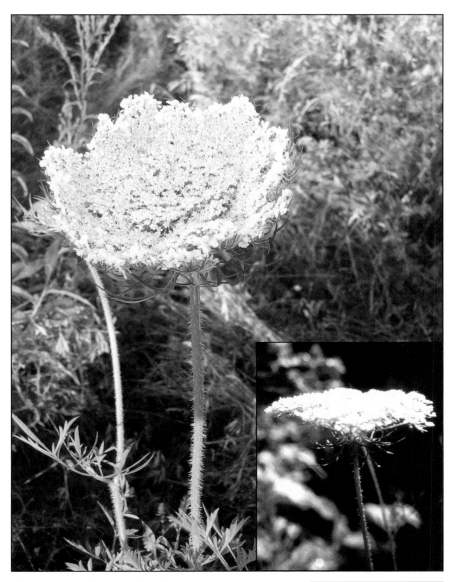

Queen Anne's Lace

Habitat: Fields, waste areas.

Characteristics: Height 18", can reach up to 24". Carrot-like odor in stem, leaves, seeds; lacy, flat-topped, umbrella-like flower clusters. Leaves are parsley-like and feathery, stems have tiny fuzz.

WARNING: PLANT IS SIMILAR TO POISONOUS LOOK-ALIKE POISON HEMLOCK. Always crush and sniff for carrot smell and look for the characteristic stem hairs for identification.

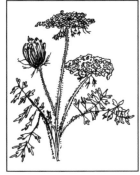

42

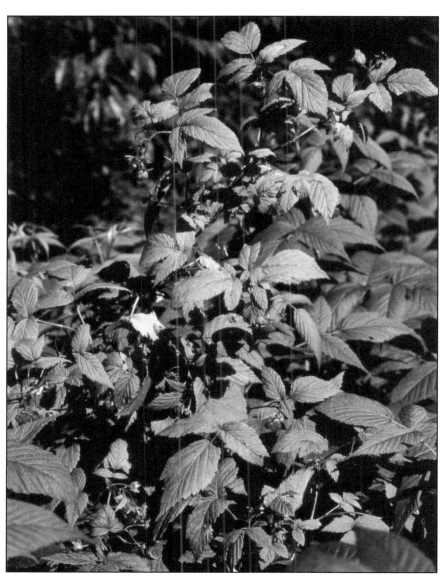

Raspberry

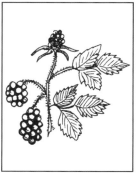

Habitat: Roadsides, rocky fields, thickets.

Characteristics: Vines average to 5' high, saw-toothed leaves in groups of 3. Round, usually red stem has prickers and white powder, fruit pebbly and red when ripe.

WARNING: Red-tinged, mature leaves may be toxic. Use only young green leaves.

43

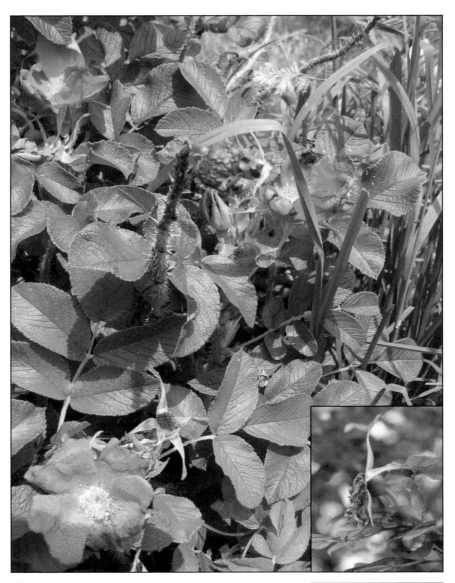

Rose

Habitat: Meadows, fields, woods, and coastal beaches.

Characteristics: There are many varieties from vines to large bushes, all of which have briars. Stems are thorny, flowers have 5-petals and in colors of yellow, pink, red or purple. Fruit is called *rose hips* and has prominent calyx lobes.

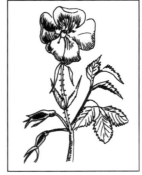

44

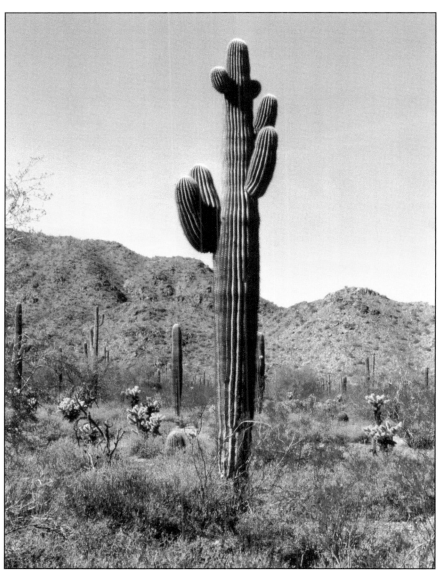

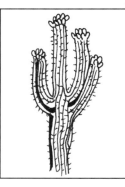

Saguaro

Habitat: Desert, rocky, gravel soil; hills, canyons, dry washes.

Characteristics: Tree-like cactus usually having 1 or more rounded arms extending branch-like from a single, thick trunk. Large, thick grooves run laterally on all parts; thick fish-hook barbs on all sides.

45

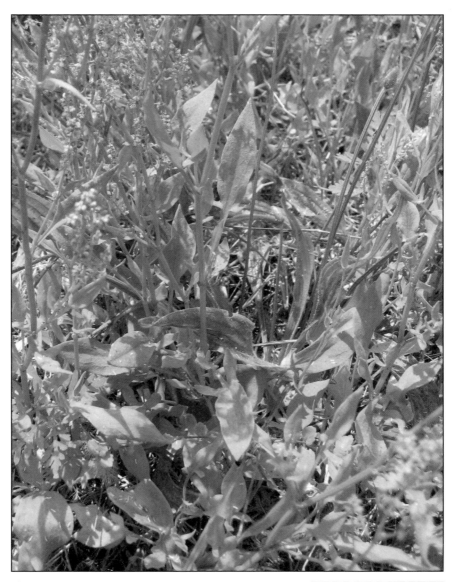

Sheep Sorrel

<u>Habitat</u>: Waste areas, roadsides.

<u>Characteristics</u>: Reddish-tinged, grassy tops, arrow-shaped leaves, tiny flowers. Mature seeds grow in spreading areas.

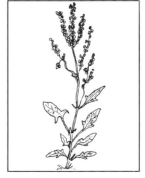

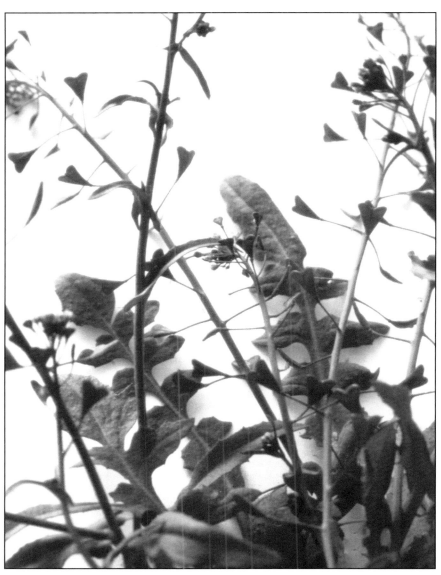

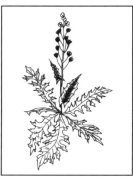

Shepherd's Purse

Habitat: Waste areas, roadsides.

Characteristics: Height is 3" to 1 1/2' high. Slender stem comes up from a spreading rosette of leaves formed flat on the ground. Leaves are deeply lobed, flower petals are 1/8" to 1/2" long; seeds resemble upside down hearts.

47

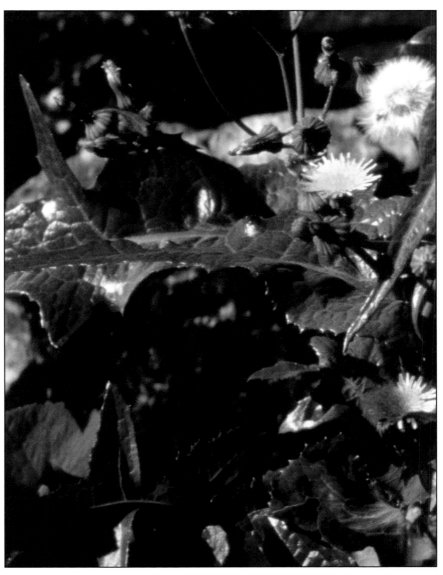

Sow Thistle

Habitat: Waste areas, roadsides, damp fields.

Characteristics: Deeply lobed leaves from a central stem on the ground, clasping around stalk to a sharp point like a sow's ear; yellow flower at the end of branch. White milk exudes from any broken part of the plant. After going to seed, a white puff ball appears with single seeds on the end of the fluff like a small dandelion.

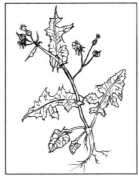

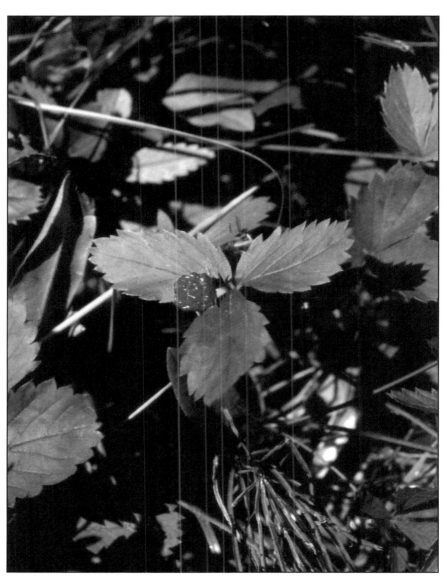

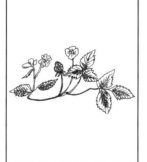

Strawberry

Habitat: Fields, roadsides, meadows.

Characteristics: Height 2", can reach 8" or more. Lobed, saw-toothed leaves in groups of 3; tiny heart-shaped strawberry fruits. White fur on young stem and leaf.

49

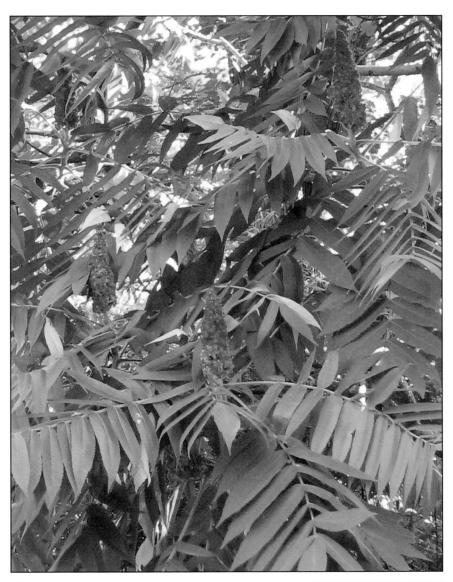

Sumac

Habitat: Field edges, roadsides.

Characteristics: A tree having smooth, dark bark with striated, raised sections; hairy stalk and twigs. Leaf fans up to 2' long, each containing 11 to 13 pairs of saw-toothed leaflets. Furry, dry red berries clustered in spires. Stems have milky sap.

WARNING: DO NOT CONFUSE WITH POISON SUMAC, WHICH HAS WHITE BERRIES.

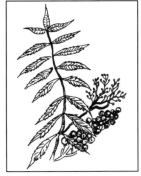

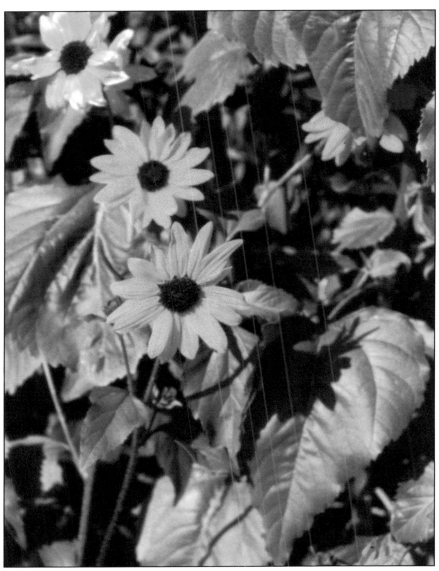

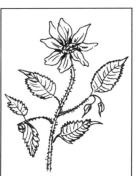

Sunflower

Habitat: Gardens, fields, sunny open areas.

Characteristics: Height 3', may reach 12' or more. Hairy stems, saw-toothed, ovate leaves, multi-petaled yellow flowers sometimes with black centers.

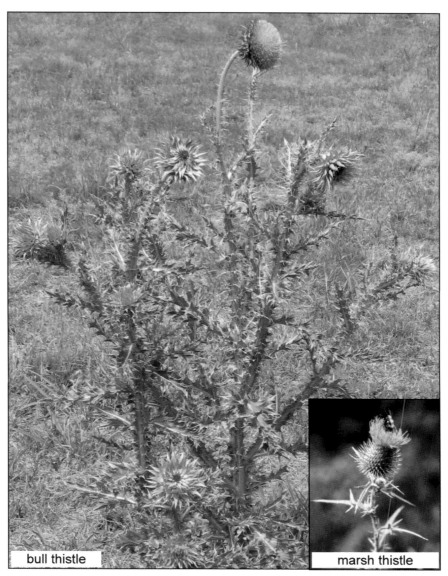

bull thistle

marsh thistle

Thistle

<u>Habitat</u>: Roadsides, fields, waste areas.

<u>Characteristics</u>: Height 2', may reach 6' or more. Leaves and stems have sharp spines (barbs) on all parts; 1 to 3 large, purplish flower heads with spines around base. There are many species, all edible.

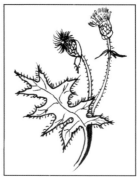

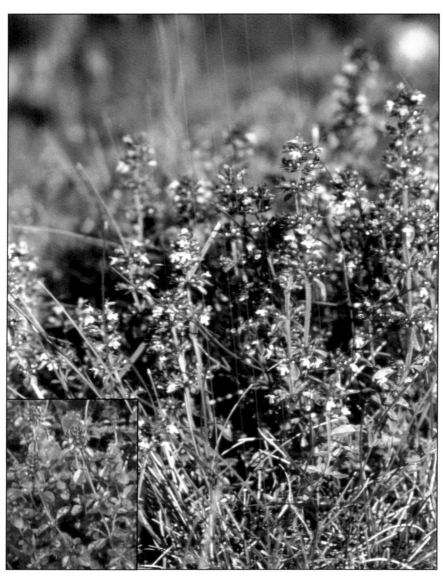

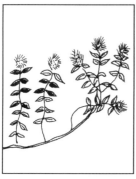

Thyme

Habitat: Roadsides, fields, waste areas.

Characteristics: Height 4" or more, grows in thick patches. Pepper-like smell, lavender spike of flowers.

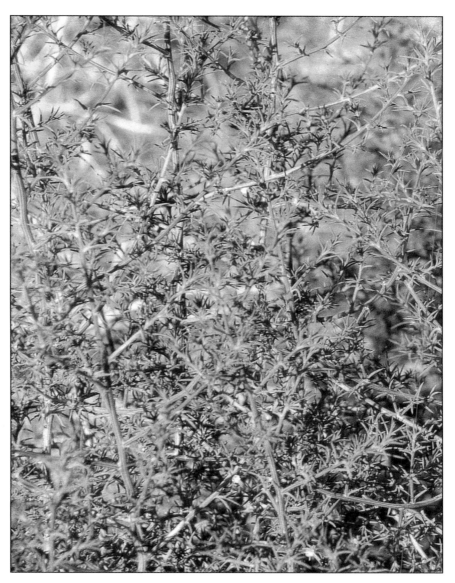

Tumbleweed

<u>Habitat</u>: Roadsides, fields, open desert, hot, dry country.

<u>Characteristics</u>: Height 2' or more; roundish prickly bush, an intricately branched plant. Often reddish with ridged stems and many tiny ends. Late in the season the plant breaks off at the base and rolls around freely in the wind, dropping its many seeds.

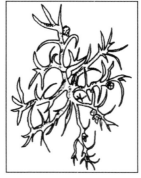

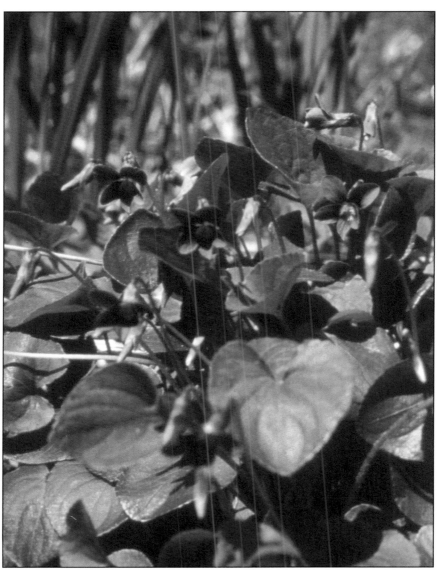

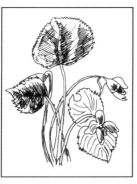

Violet

Habitat: Likes rich soil as found in moist woods, swamp sides, stream banks and damp lawns.

Characteristics: Height 4" or more; leaves vary from heart-shaped to elongated. 5-petal flowers are face-like; colors may be white, yellow, blue, or lavender. Lower petals have heavy veins and there is a "bearded" design.

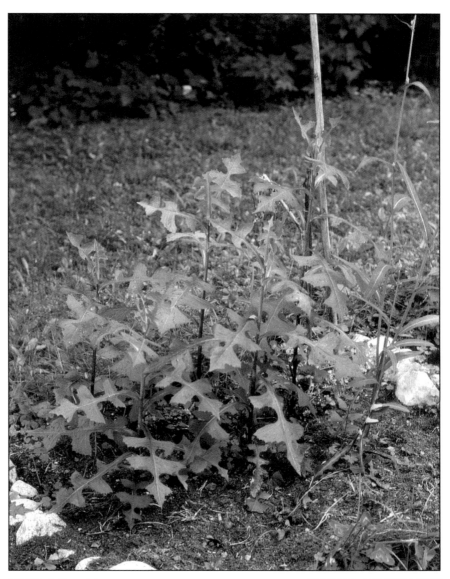

Wild Lettuce

<u>Habitat</u>: Fields, waste ground, roadsides.

<u>Characteristics</u>: Height 2' or more. Leaves are deeply lobed and irregular. Multi-branched top has many small yellow or blue blossoms. White milk exudes when any part is broken.

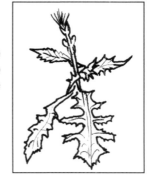

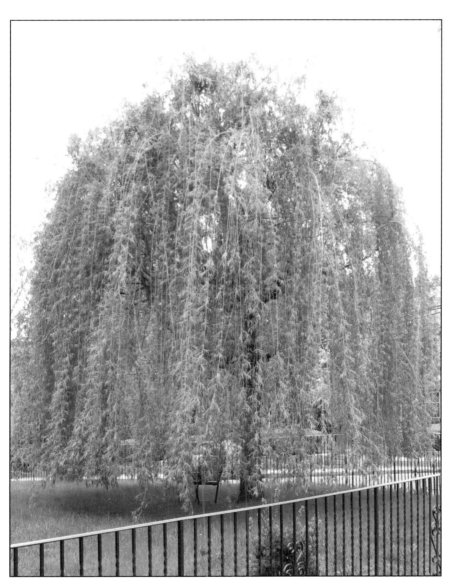

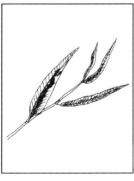

Willow

Habitat: Damp areas, stream sides and swamps.

Characteristics: Many species have drooping branches with alternate 2" leaves, short stem, sectioned twig "tendril." Flowers (catkins) are furry.

WARNING: Used sparingly for medicinal purposes. Do not ingest or use more than 10 to 12 catkins at any one time.

57

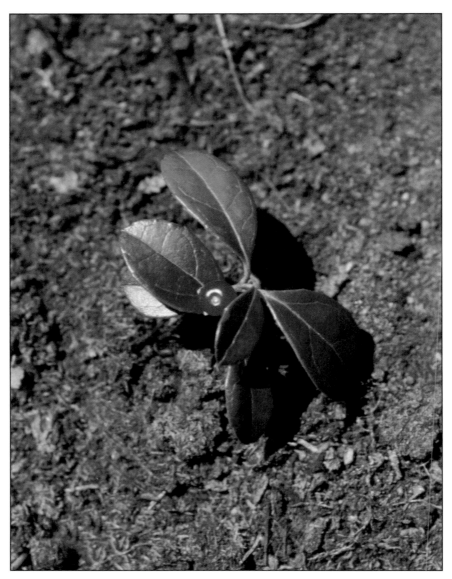

Wintergreen

<u>Habitat</u>: Wooded areas, acid soils, found under softwood trees.

<u>Characteristics</u>: Height 2" to 6" high. Flat, shiny, dark green, ovate leaves. Drooping, waxy, white flowers followed by bright red berries.

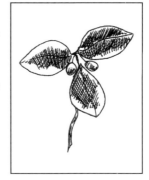

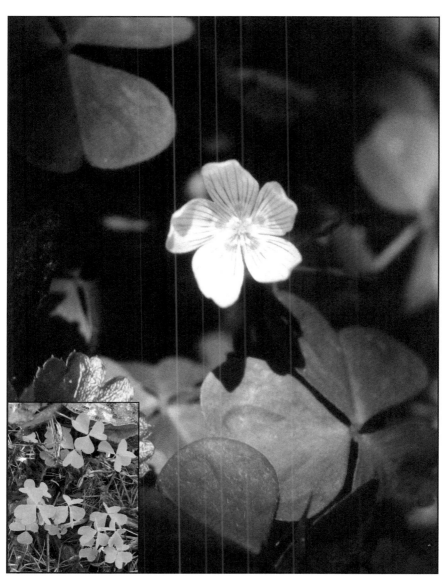

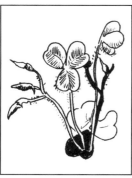

Wood Sorrel

Habitat: Fields, woods, moist places, under trees or shrubs.

Characteristics: Height 2" to 8" in bunches or carpets; leaves in 3 heart-shaped leaflets (a shamrock). Leaves have a sour lemon taste and may fold up when extremely warm or in sunshine. Flowers have 5 petals.

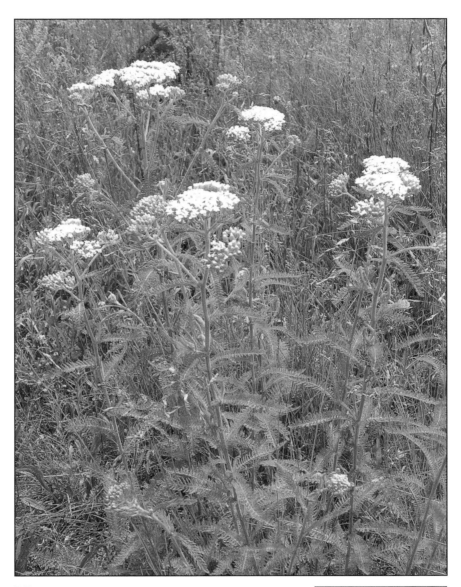

Yarrow

<u>Habitat</u>: Old fields, roadsides.

<u>Characteristics</u>: Height 16" or more; fern-like, lacy leaves which look like chipmunk's tails. White flowers have 5 petal-like rays, dozens in flat top clusters. Flowers and leaves have a slight astringent smell.

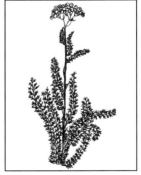

60

CPSIA information can be obtained
at www.ICGtesting.com
Printed in the USA
LVIW020825110612

285539LV00005B